# DR. BARBARA 10-DAY GREEN SMOOTHIE CLEANSE

The simple 10-day plan for mucus and full- body detox to boost immunity and reset your body and mind for optimal health and wellness

Felicia Felix

# Table of Contents

# COPYRIGHT © 2023

# CHAPTER ONE

## Introduction to Dr. Sebi's Healing Smoothies:

Dr. Sebi's healing smoothies are a part of the nutritional approach developed by Dr. Sebi, a Honduran herbalist and healer who gained prominence for his holistic approach to health and wellness. His philosophy revolves around the idea that disease is a consequence of mucus buildup in the body, primarily caused by consuming acidic and mucus-forming foods. To counteract this, Dr. Sebi advocated for an alkaline diet composed of natural, plant-based foods to cleanse the body and promote healing.

One of the key components of Dr. Sebi's dietary recommendations is the incorporation of healing smoothies. These smoothies are crafted from a selection of alkaline fruits, vegetables, and herbs, carefully chosen for their nutritional benefits and ability to support the body's natural detoxification processes. By consuming these smoothies regularly, individuals can purportedly help alkalize their bodies, reduce inflammation, and support overall health and vitality.

## Understanding Dr. Sebi's Philosophy:

Before delving into the specifics of Dr. Sebi's healing smoothies, it's essential to understand the underlying principles of his dietary philosophy. Central to his teachings is the concept of alkalinity versus acidity in the body. According to Dr. Sebi, many health issues stem from an overly acidic internal environment, which can lead to the accumulation of mucus in various organs and tissues. This acidic condition, he argues, is exacerbated by the consumption of acidic and mucus-forming foods, such as meat, dairy, refined grains, and processed foods.

In contrast, Dr. Sebi advocates for an alkaline diet primarily composed of plant-based foods. He contends that alkaline foods help to neutralize acidity in the body, reduce mucus buildup, and create an optimal environment for cellular health and regeneration. By following an alkaline diet, individuals can purportedly support the body's innate healing mechanisms and prevent or alleviate various health conditions.

## The Role of Healing Smoothies:

Healing smoothies play a crucial role in Dr. Sebi's approach to wellness by providing a concentrated source of alkaline nutrients in an easily digestible form. These smoothies typically contain a variety of alkaline fruits, such as berries, mangoes, and melons, along with leafy greens like kale, spinach, and dandelion greens. Additionally, Dr. Sebi often incorporates specific herbs and spices known for their cleansing and healing properties, such as bladderwrack, burdock root, and sarsaparilla.

The ingredients chosen for Dr. Sebi's healing smoothies are carefully selected based on their alkalinity, nutrient density, and therapeutic effects on the body. For example, leafy greens are rich in chlorophyll, a powerful antioxidant that supports detoxification and helps to oxygenate the blood. Fruits like berries and citrus fruits provide an abundance of vitamin C, which boosts the immune system and promotes collagen production for healthy skin.

**Benefits of Healing Smoothies:**

Proponents of Dr. Sebi's healing smoothies tout a wide range of potential benefits, including improved digestion, increased energy levels, clearer skin, and enhanced immune function. The alkaline nature of these smoothies is believed to help restore the body's pH balance, reducing inflammation and supporting overall vitality. Additionally, the abundance of vitamins, minerals, and phytonutrients in the ingredients may help to nourish cells, strengthen the immune system, and promote detoxification.

Some individuals also report weight loss and improved metabolic function as a result of incorporating healing smoothies into their daily routine. By replacing acidic and processed foods with nutrient-dense smoothies, individuals may naturally reduce calorie intake while still satisfying their hunger and cravings. Furthermore, the fiber content in the smoothies supports healthy digestion and helps to regulate blood sugar levels, promoting satiety and preventing energy crashes.

## Tips for Making Healing Smoothies:

Creating Dr. Sebi's healing smoothies at home is relatively simple, requiring just a few basic ingredients and a blender. To maximize the nutritional benefits, it's essential to use fresh, organic produce whenever possible. When selecting fruits and vegetables, opt for alkaline varieties such as leafy greens, berries, citrus fruits, and tropical fruits like mangoes and papayas.

In addition to fruits and vegetables, consider incorporating herbs and spices known for their cleansing and healing properties. Common additions include bladderwrack, burdock root, sarsaparilla, and sea moss. These herbs not only enhance the flavor of the smoothies but also provide additional nutritional support for detoxification and overall wellness.

To prepare a healing smoothie, simply combine your chosen ingredients in a blender with water or a nut milk of your choice. Blend until smooth and creamy, adjusting the consistency as needed by adding more liquid or ice. Feel free to experiment with different flavor combinations and ingredient ratios to suit your taste preferences and nutritional needs.

## Conclusion:

Dr. Sebi's healing smoothies are an integral part of his holistic approach to health and wellness, offering a convenient and delicious way to support the body's natural detoxification processes. By incorporating alkaline fruits, vegetables, and herbs into these smoothies, individuals can nourish their cells, reduce inflammation, and promote overall vitality. While the specific benefits of healing smoothies may vary from person to person, many individuals report improvements in digestion, energy levels, and immune function after incorporating them into their daily routine. With a focus on fresh, organic ingredients and mindful preparation, anyone can enjoy the rejuvenating benefits of Dr. Sebi's healing smoothies as part of a balanced and health-conscious lifestyle.

# CHAPTER TWO

## The Importance of Green Smoothies: Exploring Their Role in Detoxifying the Body and Boosting Nutrition

Green smoothies have gained immense popularity in recent years as a convenient and nutritious way to incorporate more greens into the diet. These vibrant concoctions typically feature a blend of leafy greens, fruits, and other wholesome ingredients, offering a powerhouse of nutrients in a refreshing and easily digestible form. Beyond their delicious taste, green smoothies are celebrated for their potential to detoxify the body and enhance overall nutrition. In this exploration, we delve into the importance of green smoothies, examining their role in detoxification and nutritional optimization.

## The Nutritional Powerhouse of Greens:

Leafy greens, such as spinach, kale, Swiss chard, and collard greens, are nutritional powerhouses packed with vitamins, minerals, antioxidants, and phytonutrients. These nutrient-dense vegetables are particularly rich in vitamins A, C, and K, as well as folate, potassium, magnesium, and calcium. They also contain a variety of beneficial plant compounds, including chlorophyll, lutein, and zeaxanthin, which have been linked to numerous health benefits.

By incorporating leafy greens into smoothies, individuals can easily increase their intake of these vital nutrients, supporting overall health and well-being. Green smoothies provide a convenient and delicious way to consume a variety of greens, allowing individuals to reap the nutritional benefits without the need for extensive meal preparation or cooking.

## Detoxification and Cleansing Properties:

Green smoothies are often touted for their detoxifying and cleansing properties, thanks to the high concentration of chlorophyll found in leafy greens. Chlorophyll is the green pigment responsible for photosynthesis in plants and has been shown to have potent detoxification effects in the body. It helps to neutralize toxins, heavy metals, and other harmful substances, promoting their elimination through the liver and kidneys.

Additionally, the fiber content in green smoothies supports healthy digestion and regularity, aiding in the removal of waste and toxins from the body. Fiber acts as a natural broom, sweeping through the digestive tract and promoting the elimination of accumulated waste material. This gentle cleansing action helps to detoxify the body and maintain optimal digestive health.

## Balanced Macronutrients for Sustained Energy:

In addition to their detoxifying properties, green smoothies provide a balanced combination of macronutrients, including carbohydrates, protein, and healthy fats, which are essential for sustained energy and overall vitality. Leafy greens are low in calories but high in fiber, making them an excellent choice for promoting satiety and preventing blood sugar spikes.

When combined with fruits, such as bananas, berries, or mangoes, green smoothies become a complete meal or snack, providing a source of carbohydrates for energy and replenishing glycogen stores. Adding sources of protein, such as Greek yogurt, tofu, or protein powder, further enhances the nutritional profile of green smoothies, supporting muscle repair and growth.

## Antioxidant Protection and Immune Support:

The fruits and vegetables used in green smoothies are rich in antioxidants, which help to neutralize harmful free radicals and protect the body from oxidative stress. Antioxidants play a critical role in supporting immune function, reducing inflammation, and preventing chronic diseases such as heart disease, cancer, and diabetes.

By regularly consuming green smoothies, individuals can bolster their antioxidant defenses and strengthen their immune system, reducing the risk of illness and promoting overall longevity. Incorporating a variety of colorful fruits and vegetables into smoothies ensures a diverse array of antioxidants, each with its unique health-promoting properties.

# Conclusion:

Green smoothies offer a myriad of benefits for detoxifying the body and boosting nutrition, making them a valuable addition to any healthy diet. Packed with leafy greens, fruits, and other wholesome ingredients, these vibrant concoctions provide a concentrated source of vitamins, minerals, antioxidants, and fiber, supporting overall health and vitality.

By regularly consuming green smoothies, individuals can detoxify their bodies, promote healthy digestion, and support immune function. With their balanced combination of macronutrients and antioxidant-rich ingredients, green smoothies offer a convenient and delicious way to nourish the body and optimize health. Whether enjoyed as a refreshing breakfast, post-workout snack, or afternoon pick-me-up, green smoothies are a simple yet powerful tool for enhancing well-being and vitality.

# CHAPTER THREE

## Dr. Barbara's Philosophy on Herbal Nutrition: Embracing Plant-Based Healing for Optimal Health

Dr. Barbara's philosophy on herbal nutrition centers around the belief that plant-based healing holds the key to achieving optimal health and wellness. Drawing inspiration from traditional herbal medicine and modern nutritional science, Dr. Barbara advocates for the incorporation of nutrient-rich herbs and botanicals into everyday diet and lifestyle practices. In this exploration, we delve into Dr. Barbara's holistic approach to herbal nutrition, highlighting the importance of embracing plant-based healing for overall well-being.

## The Healing Power of Plants:

At the core of Dr. Barbara's philosophy is the recognition of the healing power of plants. Throughout history, cultures around the world have relied on medicinal herbs and botanicals to prevent and treat various ailments. These plants contain a wealth of bioactive compounds, including vitamins, minerals, antioxidants, and phytonutrients, which exert therapeutic effects on the body.

Dr. Barbara emphasizes the importance of harnessing the inherent healing properties of plants to support overall health and vitality. By incorporating a diverse array of herbs and botanicals into the diet, individuals can nourish their bodies with essential nutrients and promote balance and harmony within.

## Nutrient Density and Bioavailability:

One of the key principles of Dr. Barbara's philosophy is the focus on nutrient density and bioavailability. Many herbs and botanicals are exceptionally rich in vitamins, minerals, and other essential nutrients, making them valuable additions to the diet. Unlike processed foods, which may be lacking in nutrients and laden with additives and preservatives, whole herbs offer a natural and potent source of nutrition.

Furthermore, the bioactive compounds found in herbs are often more readily absorbed and utilized by the body compared to synthetic supplements. Dr. Barbara emphasizes the importance of consuming herbs in their whole, unprocessed form to maximize nutrient absorption and bioavailability. This ensures that individuals can derive the greatest benefit from the nutritional properties of these plants.

## Balancing the Body's Ecosystem:

In addition to providing essential nutrients, herbs and botanicals play a crucial role in balancing the body's internal ecosystem. Many herbs possess adaptogenic properties, which help the body adapt to stress and maintain homeostasis. By supporting the body's natural regulatory mechanisms, these herbs can help alleviate symptoms of imbalance and promote overall resilience and vitality.

Dr. Barbara encourages individuals to explore the use of adaptogenic herbs such as ashwagandha, rhodiola, and holy basil to support stress management and enhance overall well-being. By incorporating these herbs into their daily routines, individuals can cultivate greater resilience to the demands of modern life and experience a heightened sense of vitality and equilibrium.

## Promoting Holistic Wellness:

Dr. Barbara's philosophy on herbal nutrition extends beyond the physical aspects of health to encompass the holistic well-being of the individual. She recognizes the interconnectedness of body, mind, and spirit and emphasizes the importance of nurturing all aspects of the self to achieve true wellness.

In addition to incorporating nutrient-rich herbs into the diet, Dr. Barbara encourages practices such as mindfulness, meditation, and self-care to promote emotional and spiritual balance. She believes that by cultivating a deep sense of connection with oneself and the natural world, individuals can unlock their innate healing potential and experience profound transformation on all levels.

**Conclusion:**

Dr. Barbara's philosophy on herbal nutrition offers a holistic approach to achieving optimal health and wellness. By embracing the healing power of plants and incorporating nutrient-rich herbs into the diet, individuals can nourish their bodies, support internal balance, and promote overall vitality. Dr. Barbara's emphasis on nutrient density, bioavailability, and holistic wellness serves as a guiding framework for those seeking to harness the transformative potential of plant-based healing for greater health and vitality.

# CHAPTER FOUR

## Understanding Detoxification: Insights into the Body's Natural Cleansing Processes and How Green Smoothies Support Them

Detoxification is a vital physiological process through which the body eliminates toxins and harmful substances to maintain health and well-being. While the body has its built-in detoxification mechanisms, various lifestyle factors, including poor diet, environmental pollutants, and stress, can overwhelm these processes, leading to toxin buildup and potential health issues. In this exploration, we delve into the body's natural cleansing processes, the importance of detoxification, and how green smoothies can support these mechanisms.

### The Body's Natural Detoxification Processes:

The human body is equipped with several organs and systems that play key roles in detoxification. The liver is the primary organ responsible for processing toxins and metabolic waste products, converting them into less harmful substances that can be excreted from the body. Additionally, the kidneys filter waste products from the blood and eliminate them through urine, while the lymphatic system helps remove toxins and cellular waste from tissues.

Other organs involved in detoxification include the lungs, which expel toxins through respiration, and the skin, which eliminates waste products through sweat. Together, these organs work synergistically to rid the body of harmful substances and maintain internal balance.

**Challenges to Detoxification:**

Despite the body's remarkable detoxification capabilities, modern lifestyles characterized by processed foods, environmental pollutants, and chronic stress can overwhelm these processes, leading to toxin accumulation. Poor dietary choices, in particular, can burden the liver and other detoxification organs, hindering their ability to effectively neutralize and eliminate toxins.

Toxins that accumulate in the body can disrupt cellular function, impair immune function, and contribute to the development of chronic diseases such as obesity, diabetes, and cardiovascular disease. Therefore, supporting the body's natural detoxification processes is essential for overall health and well-being.

## The Role of Green Smoothies in Detoxification:

Green smoothies offer a convenient and effective way to support the body's natural detoxification processes. Packed with leafy greens, fruits, and other nutrient-rich ingredients, green smoothies provide a concentrated source of vitamins, minerals, antioxidants, and fiber that promote detoxification and overall health.

Leafy greens such as spinach, kale, and Swiss chard are particularly rich in chlorophyll, a green pigment with potent detoxifying properties. Chlorophyll helps neutralize toxins, support liver function, and promote the elimination of waste products from the body. Additionally, the fiber content in green smoothies supports healthy digestion and regular bowel movements, facilitating the removal of toxins from the gastrointestinal tract.

## Nutrient-Rich Ingredients for Cellular Health:

In addition to chlorophyll, green smoothies contain a variety of other nutrients that support cellular health and detoxification. Fruits such as berries, apples, and citrus fruits provide antioxidants such as vitamin C and flavonoids, which help protect cells from oxidative damage and promote detoxification.

Furthermore, green smoothies often include ingredients such as ginger, turmeric, and cilantro, which possess anti-inflammatory and antioxidant properties that support detoxification and overall well-being. These herbs and spices not only enhance the flavor of green smoothies but also provide additional therapeutic benefits for the body.

## Hydration and Electrolyte Balance:

Proper hydration is essential for supporting detoxification processes, as it helps flush toxins from the body and maintain optimal cellular function. Green smoothies, which are typically made with water or a liquid base such as coconut water or almond milk, help keep the body hydrated and support detoxification.

Additionally, ingredients such as coconut water provide electrolytes such as potassium and magnesium, which are crucial for maintaining fluid balance and supporting cellular detoxification. By staying hydrated and replenishing electrolytes with green smoothies, individuals can support their body's natural detoxification processes and promote overall health and well-being.

## Conclusion:

Detoxification is a fundamental process that allows the body to eliminate toxins and maintain internal balance. While the body has its built-in detoxification mechanisms, various lifestyle factors can hinder these processes, leading to toxin accumulation and potential health issues. Green smoothies offer a convenient and effective way to support the body's natural detoxification processes by providing a concentrated source of nutrients, antioxidants, and fiber that promote detoxification and overall health. By incorporating green smoothies into their diets regularly, individuals can support their body's natural detoxification processes, promote cellular health, and enhance overall well-being.

# CHAPTER FIVE

## Selecting the Right Ingredients: Identifying Key Greens and Herbs for Detoxifying Smoothies

When creating detoxifying smoothies, selecting the right ingredients is crucial to maximize their effectiveness in supporting the body's natural cleansing processes. Incorporating nutrient-rich greens and herbs can enhance the detoxification potential of smoothies, providing a wealth of vitamins, minerals, antioxidants, and phytonutrients. In this guide, we explore key greens and herbs that are ideal for detoxifying smoothies, highlighting their unique benefits and how they contribute to overall health and well-being.

**Leafy Greens:**

Leafy greens are the foundation of detoxifying smoothies, providing a wealth of essential nutrients and phytochemicals that support the body's natural detoxification processes. Some key greens to consider including in detoxifying smoothies are:

1. **Spinach:** Spinach is a nutritional powerhouse rich in vitamins A, C, and K, as well as folate, iron, and magnesium. It also contains chlorophyll, which helps to alkalize the body and support detoxification.

2. **Kale:** Kale is another nutrient-dense green packed with vitamins, minerals, and antioxidants. It is particularly rich in

vitamin K, which supports liver function and blood clotting, as well as glucosinolates, compounds that aid in detoxification.

3. **Swiss Chard:** Swiss chard is high in antioxidants, including vitamin C and beta-carotene, which help protect cells from oxidative damage. It also contains fiber, which supports healthy digestion and detoxification.

4. **Dandelion Greens:** Dandelion greens are known for their liver-cleansing properties and are rich in vitamins A, C, and K, as well as calcium and iron. They stimulate bile production, which aids in the digestion of fats and the elimination of toxins.

5. **Cilantro:** Cilantro is a flavorful herb that helps to remove heavy metals from the body, making it an excellent addition to detoxifying smoothies. It also contains antioxidants and anti-inflammatory compounds that support overall health.

**Herbs and Spices:**

In addition to leafy greens, herbs and spices can further enhance the detoxification potential of smoothies by providing additional therapeutic benefits. Some key herbs and spices to consider incorporating into detoxifying smoothies include:

1. **Parsley:** Parsley is a natural diuretic that helps flush excess water and toxins from the body. It is also rich in vitamins A,

C, and K, as well as chlorophyll, which supports detoxification and alkalizes the body.

2. **Ginger:** Ginger has anti-inflammatory and digestive properties that support detoxification and improve digestion. It also aids in the elimination of toxins by promoting sweating and stimulating circulation.

3. **Turmeric:** Turmeric contains curcumin, a potent antioxidant and anti-inflammatory compound that supports detoxification and liver health. It also aids in digestion and helps reduce inflammation throughout the body.

4. **Mint:** Mint has a refreshing flavor and contains menthol, which helps soothe the digestive tract and promote healthy digestion. It also has mild detoxifying properties and can help alleviate bloating and gas.

5. **Cinnamon:** Cinnamon helps regulate blood sugar levels and improve insulin sensitivity, which supports overall health and detoxification. It also has anti-inflammatory and antimicrobial properties that promote digestive health.

**Conclusion:**

Incorporating key greens, herbs, and spices into detoxifying smoothies can enhance their effectiveness in supporting the body's natural cleansing processes. Leafy greens provide essential nutrients and chlorophyll that alkalize the body and support detoxification, while herbs and spices offer additional therapeutic benefits such as anti-inflammatory and digestive support. By selecting the right ingredients and combining them in delicious and nutrient-rich smoothies, individuals can support their body's detoxification efforts and promote overall health and well-being.

# CHAPTER SIX

## Creating Delicious and Nutrient-Packed Smoothie Recipes: Step-by-Step Instructions for Blending

Blending nutrient-packed smoothies at home is a fantastic way to incorporate essential vitamins, minerals, and antioxidants into your diet while enjoying delicious flavors. Whether you're aiming to support detoxification, boost energy levels, or simply nourish your body with wholesome ingredients, creating smoothies is easy and customizable. In this guide, I'll provide step-by-step instructions for blending delicious and nutrient-packed smoothie recipes that will leave you feeling refreshed and revitalized.

**Step 1: Gather Your Ingredients:**

Start by gathering all the ingredients you'll need for your smoothie recipe. This typically includes a combination of leafy greens, fruits, liquid base, protein source (optional), and any additional add-ins such as herbs, spices, or superfoods. Here's a basic breakdown of common smoothie ingredients:

- Leafy Greens: Spinach, kale, Swiss chard, or dandelion greens.

- Fruits: Berries, bananas, mangoes, apples, or citrus fruits.

- Liquid Base: Water, coconut water, almond milk, or coconut milk.

- Protein Source: Greek yogurt, tofu, protein powder, or nut butter (optional).

- Add-Ins: Herbs (mint, parsley), spices (ginger, cinnamon), superfoods (chia seeds, flaxseeds), or sweeteners (honey, dates).

**Step 2: Prepare Your Ingredients:**

Wash and chop your fruits and vegetables as needed, removing any stems, seeds, or tough parts. If you're using frozen fruits, you can skip this step. Measure out your desired quantities of each ingredient based on your recipe or personal preferences.

**Step 3: Assemble Your Blender:**

Assemble your blender and make sure it's clean and ready to use. Add the ingredients to the blender in the following order:

1. Liquid Base: Pour in your chosen liquid base to help facilitate blending and achieve your desired consistency. Start with about 1/2 to 1 cup, depending on the size of your smoothie and your preference for thickness.

2. Leafy Greens: Add your leafy greens next, followed by any additional vegetables or herbs you're using.

3. Fruits: Add your fruits on top of the greens, ensuring that they are evenly distributed throughout the blender.

4. Protein Source and Add-Ins: If you're including a protein source or any additional add-ins, add them on top of the fruits.

**Step 4: Blend Until Smooth:**

Secure the lid of your blender tightly and start blending on low speed, gradually increasing to high speed. Blend the ingredients for about 30 seconds to 1 minute, or until the mixture is smooth and creamy. If necessary, pause and scrape down the sides of the blender with a spatula to ensure all ingredients are incorporated.

**Step 5: Taste and Adjust:**

Once blended, taste your smoothie and adjust the flavor and consistency as needed. You can add more liquid if the smoothie is too thick, or additional fruits or sweeteners if it needs more sweetness. For a thicker consistency, add ice cubes or frozen fruits and blend again until smooth.

**Step 6: Serve and Enjoy:**

Pour your freshly blended smoothie into glasses or bowls and garnish with additional toppings if desired. Serve immediately and enjoy your delicious and nutrient-packed creation!

**Conclusion:**

Creating delicious and nutrient-packed smoothie recipes at home is a simple and rewarding process. By following these step-by-step instructions and experimenting with different combinations of ingredients, you can whip up a variety of smoothies to suit your taste preferences and nutritional needs. Whether enjoyed as a quick breakfast, post-workout snack, or refreshing pick-me-up, homemade smoothies are a convenient and delicious way to nourish your body and support overall health and well-being.

# CHAPTER SEVEN

# Supporting the Body's Elimination Pathways: How Dr. Barbara's Smoothie Cleanse Enhances Detox Processes

Dr. Barbara's Smoothie Cleanse is a holistic approach to detoxification that focuses on supporting the body's natural elimination pathways to remove toxins and waste products effectively. By incorporating nutrient-rich ingredients into smoothies, this cleanse provides essential vitamins, minerals, antioxidants, and fiber that promote detoxification and overall well-being. In this guide, we'll explore how Dr. Barbara's Smoothie Cleanse enhances the body's detox processes by supporting key elimination pathways.

## 1. Liver Support:

The liver plays a central role in detoxification by metabolizing and neutralizing toxins before they can harm the body. Dr. Barbara's Smoothie Cleanse includes ingredients such as leafy greens, beets, and dandelion root, which support liver health and function. These ingredients contain compounds that stimulate bile production, enhance liver detoxification pathways, and promote the elimination of toxins from the body.

Leafy greens such as spinach and kale are rich in chlorophyll, a green pigment with potent detoxifying properties. Chlorophyll helps to neutralize toxins and support liver function, making it an essential component of the smoothie cleanse. Additionally, beets contain betalains, antioxidants that support liver detoxification and help protect against oxidative damage.

## 2. Kidney Support:

The kidneys filter waste products and toxins from the blood, excreting them through urine. Dr. Barbara's Smoothie Cleanse includes ingredients such as cucumber, celery, and parsley, which support kidney health and function. These ingredients have diuretic properties that help flush toxins from the kidneys and promote urine production.

Cucumber and celery are both hydrating and low in calories, making them excellent choices for supporting kidney health during the cleanse. Parsley is rich in antioxidants and has diuretic properties that support kidney function and promote the elimination of toxins.

## 3. Digestive Support:

A healthy digestive system is essential for effective detoxification, as it ensures the proper breakdown, absorption, and elimination of nutrients and waste products. Dr. Barbara's Smoothie Cleanse includes ingredients such as fiber-rich fruits, vegetables, and herbs that support digestive health and regularity.

Fruits such as berries, apples, and bananas are rich in fiber, which helps promote healthy digestion and regular bowel movements. Additionally, herbs such as ginger, mint, and fennel have digestive properties that help soothe the digestive tract, reduce bloating, and alleviate gas.

## 4. Lymphatic Support:

The lymphatic system plays a crucial role in detoxification by removing toxins and waste products from the body's tissues and transporting them to the bloodstream for elimination. Dr. Barbara's Smoothie Cleanse includes ingredients such as citrus fruits, berries, and leafy greens, which support lymphatic health and function.

Citrus fruits such as lemons, limes, and oranges are rich in vitamin C and antioxidants that support lymphatic drainage and help remove toxins from the body. Berries are also high in antioxidants and contain compounds that support lymphatic function and promote detoxification.

## Conclusion:

Dr. Barbara's Smoothie Cleanse enhances the body's detox processes by supporting key elimination pathways, including the liver, kidneys, digestive system, and lymphatic system. By incorporating nutrient-rich ingredients into smoothies, this cleanse provides essential nutrients and compounds that promote detoxification, remove toxins, and support overall health and well-being. Whether used as a short-term cleanse or incorporated into a long-term wellness routine, Dr. Barbara's Smoothie Cleanse offers a holistic approach to detoxification that nourishes the body and supports optimal health.

# CHAPTER EIGHT

## Preparing for the Cleanse: Guidelines for Pre-Cleanse Preparation and Transitioning to Smoothie-Based Nutrition

Embarking on a cleanse, such as Dr. Barbara's Smoothie Cleanse, requires thoughtful preparation to maximize its effectiveness and ensure a smooth transition to a smoothie-based diet. Preparing the body beforehand and gradually transitioning to a smoothie-based nutrition plan can help minimize potential detox symptoms and optimize the benefits of the cleanse. In this guide, we'll outline guidelines for pre-cleanse preparation and transitioning to smoothie-based nutrition to help you embark on your cleanse journey with confidence.

## 1. Pre-Cleanse Preparation:

Before starting the cleanse, it's essential to prepare your body by gradually eliminating processed foods, caffeine, alcohol, and refined sugars from your diet. Here are some pre-cleanse preparation guidelines to follow:

- **Hydrate:** Drink plenty of water to stay hydrated and support your body's detoxification processes.

- **Increase Plant Foods:** Incorporate more fruits, vegetables, whole grains, and legumes into your diet to increase your intake of fiber, vitamins, and minerals.

- **Reduce Toxins:** Avoid exposure to environmental toxins as much as possible by choosing organic produce, using natural cleaning products, and avoiding plastics and synthetic chemicals.

- **Limit Stimulants:** Gradually reduce your intake of caffeine and alcohol to minimize withdrawal symptoms during the cleanse.

- **Get Adequate Sleep:** Aim for 7-9 hours of quality sleep per night to support your body's natural detoxification and regeneration processes.

## 2. Transitioning to Smoothie-Based Nutrition:

Transitioning to a smoothie-based nutrition plan before starting the cleanse can help prepare your body and ease the transition. Here's how to transition effectively:

- **Start Slowly:** Begin by incorporating one smoothie into your daily routine as a meal replacement or snack. Choose nutrient-dense ingredients such as leafy greens, fruits, and protein sources to maximize nutritional intake.

- **Gradually Increase Frequency:** Gradually increase the number of smoothies you consume each day, replacing one or two meals with smoothies while still eating whole foods for the remainder of your meals.

- **Experiment with Ingredients:** Use this time to experiment with different smoothie recipes and ingredients to find combinations that you enjoy and that meet your nutritional needs.

- **Listen to Your Body:** Pay attention to how your body responds to the increased intake of fruits, vegetables, and liquids. Adjust your smoothie recipes and portion sizes as needed based on your energy levels, digestion, and overall well-being.

## 3. Preparing for the Cleanse:

As you approach the start date of the cleanse, take time to prepare mentally and physically for the journey ahead. Here are some final steps to prepare for the cleanse:

- **Set Intentions:** Take a moment to reflect on your reasons for doing the cleanse and set intentions for what you hope to achieve. Visualize success and commit to honoring your body throughout the process.

- **Stock Up on Supplies:** Ensure you have all the necessary ingredients and equipment for making smoothies, including a high-quality blender, fresh fruits and vegetables, leafy greens, and any additional add-ins or supplements recommended for the cleanse.

- **Clear Your Schedule:** Try to minimize stress and obligations during the cleanse period by clearing your schedule as much as possible. Allow yourself time for rest, relaxation, and self-care activities to support the detoxification process.

- **Stay Flexible:** Be open to adjusting your plan as needed based on how your body responds to the cleanse. Listen to your body's cues and make modifications as necessary to ensure a safe and successful experience.

**Conclusion:**

Preparation is key to a successful cleanse experience. By following these guidelines for pre-cleanse preparation and transitioning to smoothie-based nutrition, you can set yourself up for a smooth and effective cleanse journey. Remember to approach the cleanse with patience, mindfulness, and self-compassion, and trust in your body's ability to heal and rejuvenate through the process.

# CHAPTER NINE

# Testimonials of Transformation: Inspiring Stories of Individuals Who Have Benefited from Dr. Barbara's Cleanse

Dr. Barbara's Cleanse has touched the lives of many individuals seeking to improve their health and well-being through holistic nutrition and detoxification. These inspiring stories of transformation showcase the profound impact that the cleanse has had on individuals' lives, from improved energy levels and digestion to enhanced mental clarity and overall vitality. In this collection of testimonials, we celebrate the journeys of those who have experienced positive changes through Dr. Barbara's Cleanse.

**1. Sarah's Journey to Vibrant Health:**

"I had been struggling with low energy and digestive issues for years when I decided to try Dr. Barbara's Cleanse. Within just a few days of starting the cleanse, I noticed a remarkable difference in my energy levels and digestion. I felt lighter, more alert, and more vibrant than I had in years. The smoothies were delicious and satisfying, and I loved knowing that I was nourishing my body with wholesome ingredients. After completing the cleanse, I continued to incorporate smoothies into my daily routine, and I've never felt better. Thank you, Dr. Barbara, for helping me reclaim my health and vitality!"

**2. Mark's Renewed Sense of Well-Being:**

"After years of struggling with weight gain, fatigue, and digestive issues, I was feeling hopeless about ever feeling healthy again. That's when I discovered Dr. Barbara's Cleanse. I was skeptical at first, but after just one week on the cleanse, I was amazed by the changes I experienced. Not only did I lose weight and gain energy, but my digestion improved, and I felt a renewed sense of well-being. The cleanse helped me break free from unhealthy eating habits and reset my body's natural balance. I'm grateful to Dr. Barbara for creating such an effective and life-changing program."

**3. Emily's Journey to Self-Discovery:**

"Dr. Barbara's Cleanse was more than just a physical detox for me—it was a journey of self-discovery and transformation. As someone who struggled with emotional eating and poor body image, I found solace in the nourishing and healing power of the cleanse. The smoothies provided me with a sense of comfort and satisfaction that I had never experienced with other diets. Through the cleanse, I learned to listen to my body's cues, nourish myself with love and compassion, and embrace a healthier relationship with food. I am forever grateful to Dr. Barbara for guiding me on this journey of healing and self-discovery."

**4. Michael's Path to Optimal Health:**

"For years, I had been struggling with chronic health issues, including inflammation, joint pain, and fatigue. Conventional treatments offered little relief, so I turned to Dr. Barbara's Cleanse as a last resort. I was amazed by the results. Not only did my symptoms improve significantly, but I also experienced a newfound sense of vitality and well-being. The cleanse helped me identify food sensitivities and adopt a healthier lifestyle that supports my body's natural healing processes. I'm thrilled to say that I'm now living pain-free and enjoying life to the fullest, thanks to Dr. Barbara's transformative cleanse."

**Conclusion:**

These testimonials offer a glimpse into the profound impact that Dr. Barbara's Cleanse has had on the lives of individuals seeking to improve their health and well-being. From increased energy and vitality to improved digestion and emotional well-being, the cleanse has empowered countless individuals to reclaim their health and vitality. These inspiring stories serve as a testament to the transformative power of holistic nutrition and detoxification and the profound difference it can make in one's life.

# CHAPTER TEN

## Post-Cleanse Maintenance: Strategies for Sustaining Health and Wellness Through Long-Term Dietary and Lifestyle Changes

Completing a cleanse, such as Dr. Barbara's Cleanse, marks the beginning of a journey toward sustained health and wellness. While the cleanse provides a powerful reset for the body, maintaining the benefits over the long term requires ongoing commitment to healthy dietary and lifestyle practices. In this guide, we'll explore strategies for post-cleanse maintenance, including dietary modifications, lifestyle changes, and supportive habits to help you sustain health and wellness for the long term.

**1. Embrace a Whole Foods Diet:**

Transitioning to a whole foods diet rich in fruits, vegetables, lean proteins, and whole grains is essential for sustaining the benefits of the cleanse. Focus on incorporating nutrient-dense foods into your meals and minimizing processed foods, refined sugars, and artificial additives. Choose organic, locally sourced, and seasonal produce whenever possible to maximize nutritional value and minimize exposure to pesticides and toxins.

**2. Maintain Hydration:**

Proper hydration is key to supporting overall health and detoxification processes. Continue to drink plenty of water throughout the day to stay hydrated and flush toxins from the body. Aim for at least eight glasses of water per day, and consider incorporating hydrating foods such as fruits, vegetables, and herbal teas into your diet to support hydration.

## 3. Prioritize Sleep and Stress Management:

Quality sleep and stress management are vital components of maintaining health and wellness. Aim for 7-9 hours of restful sleep per night to support cellular repair, hormone regulation, and cognitive function. Practice stress-reducing techniques such as meditation, deep breathing, yoga, or mindfulness to promote relaxation and balance in your daily life.

## 4. Incorporate Regular Physical Activity:

Regular physical activity is essential for supporting overall health, metabolism, and detoxification processes. Aim for at least 30 minutes of moderate-intensity exercise most days of the week, such as brisk walking, cycling, swimming, or yoga. Find activities that you enjoy and make them a regular part of your routine to promote cardiovascular health, muscle strength, and flexibility.

## 5. Practice Mindful Eating:

Mindful eating involves paying attention to the sensory experience of eating and tuning into hunger and fullness cues. Take time to savor and enjoy your meals, chew slowly, and listen to your body's signals of hunger and satiety. Avoid distractions such as television, computers, or smartphones while eating, and cultivate gratitude for the nourishment your food provides.

## 6. Continue to Support Detoxification:

Supporting the body's natural detoxification processes is essential for maintaining health and wellness over the long term. Incorporate detoxifying foods such as leafy greens, cruciferous vegetables, herbs, and spices into your meals regularly. Consider periodic cleanses or detox protocols to give your body an extra boost and remove accumulated toxins.

## 7. Cultivate a Supportive Environment:

Surround yourself with a supportive environment that encourages healthy habits and positive lifestyle choices. Seek out like-minded individuals who share your commitment to health and wellness, and engage in activities that nourish your body, mind, and spirit. Create a home environment that supports your dietary and lifestyle goals, with plenty of healthy foods, opportunities for physical activity, and spaces for relaxation and self-care.

## Conclusion:

Maintaining health and wellness after completing a cleanse requires ongoing commitment to healthy dietary and lifestyle practices. By embracing a whole foods diet, prioritizing hydration, sleep, and stress management, incorporating regular physical activity, practicing mindful eating, supporting detoxification, and cultivating a supportive environment, you can sustain the benefits of the cleanse and continue to thrive in the long term. Remember that small, consistent changes over time can lead to significant improvements in your health and well-being, so be patient and compassionate with yourself as you embark on this journey of lasting transformation.

# BONUS: SOME ESSENTIAL HERBAL REMEDIES TO KNOW

**Ashwagandha:**

**Definition:** Ashwagandha, scientifically known as Withaniasomnifera, is a small shrub native to India, the Middle East, and parts of Africa. It has a long history of use in Ayurvedic medicine for its potential health benefits, particularly for its adaptogenic properties.

**Ingredients:** Ashwagandha root contains various bioactive compounds, including alkaloids (such as withanolides), steroidal lactones, and flavonoids. These compounds are believed to contribute to the herb's medicinal properties, including its potential as an adaptogen, anti-inflammatory, and immune-modulating agent.

**How to Prepare:** Ashwagandha is typically consumed as a powdered root, herbal tea, tincture, or in supplement form (such as capsules or tablets). To make tea, dried ashwagandha root is steeped in hot water for several minutes before being strained and consumed.

**Dosage:** The appropriate dosage of ashwagandha can vary depending on factors such as age, health status, and the specific preparation being used. It's important to follow the recommended dosage on the product label or consult with a qualified herbalist or healthcare professional for personalized guidance.

**How to Use:** Ashwagandha powder, tea, tincture, or supplements are typically taken orally. It's often consumed to support stress management, promote relaxation, and boost overall vitality and well-being.

**Side Effects:** Ashwagandha is generally considered safe for most people when used in moderate amounts. However, some individuals may experience mild side effects such as gastrointestinal upset or drowsiness. It may also interact with certain medications or have adverse effects in individuals with certain health conditions, such as autoimmune diseases or thyroid disorders. Pregnant or breastfeeding individuals should consult with a healthcare professional before using ashwagandha supplements. It's important to use ashwagandha under the guidance of a healthcare professional and to discontinue use if any adverse effects occur.

**Astragalus:**

**Definition:** Astragalus, scientifically known as Astragalus membranaceus, is a flowering plant native to China and Mongolia but also found in other parts of Asia. It has been used for centuries in traditional Chinese medicine for its potential health benefits, particularly for its immune-enhancing properties.

**Ingredients:** Astragalus root contains various bioactive compounds, including polysaccharides, saponins (such as astragalosides), flavonoids, and amino acids. These compounds are believed to contribute to the herb's medicinal properties, including its potential as an adaptogen, immunomodulator, and anti-inflammatory agent.

**How to Prepare:** Astragalus is typically consumed as a powdered root, herbal tea, tincture, or in supplement form (such as capsules or tablets). To make tea, dried astragalus root slices are simmered in water for several minutes before being strained and consumed.

**Dosage:** The appropriate dosage of astragalus can vary depending on factors such as age, health status, and the specific preparation being used. It's important to follow the recommended dosage on the product label or consult with a qualified herbalist or healthcare professional for personalized guidance.

**How to Use:** Astragalus powder, tea, tincture, or supplements are typically taken orally. It's often consumed to support immune function, promote vitality, and enhance overall well-being.

**Side Effects:** Astragalus is generally considered safe for most people when used in moderate amounts. However, some individuals may experience mild side effects such as gastrointestinal upset or allergic reactions. It may also interact with certain medications or have adverse effects in individuals with certain health conditions, such as autoimmune diseases or diabetes. Pregnant or breastfeeding individuals should consult with a healthcare professional before using astragalus supplements. It's important to use astragalus under the guidance of a healthcare professional and to discontinue use if any adverse effects occur.

**Black Cohosh:**

**Definition:** Black cohosh, scientifically known as Actaea racemosa (formerly Cimicifuga racemosa), is a perennial herb native to North America. It has a long history of use in traditional Native American medicine and later in folk medicine for its potential health benefits, particularly for women's health.

**Ingredients:** Black cohosh root contains various bioactive compounds, including triterpene glycosides (such as actein and cimicifugoside), phenolic acids, and flavonoids. These compounds are believed to contribute to the herb's medicinal properties, including its potential as a hormone-balancing agent and its ability to relieve menopausal symptoms.

**How to Prepare:** Black cohosh is typically consumed as a powdered root, herbal tea, tincture, or in supplement form (such as capsules or tablets). To make tea, dried black cohosh root is steeped in hot water for several minutes before being strained and consumed.

**Dosage:** The appropriate dosage of black cohosh can vary depending on factors such as age, health status, and the specific preparation being used. It's important to follow the recommended dosage on the product label or consult with a qualified herbalist or healthcare professional for personalized guidance.

**How to Use:** Black cohosh powder, tea, tincture, or supplements are typically taken orally. It's often used by women to support hormonal balance, relieve menopausal symptoms such as hot flashes and night sweats, and promote overall well-being.

**Side Effects:** Black cohosh is generally considered safe for most people when used in moderate amounts. However, some individuals may experience mild side effects such as gastrointestinal upset or allergic reactions. It may also interact with certain medications or have adverse effects in individuals with certain health conditions, such as liver disease or hormone-sensitive conditions. Pregnant or breastfeeding individuals should consult with a healthcare professional before using black cohosh supplements. It's important to use black cohosh under the guidance of a healthcare professional and to discontinue use if any adverse effects occur.

**Blessed Thistle:**

**Definition:** Blessed thistle, scientifically known as Cnicusbenedictus, is an annual or biennial herb native to the

Mediterranean region but also found in other parts of Europe, Asia, and North Africa. It has been used historically in traditional medicine for its potential health benefits, particularly for digestive and liver health.

**Ingredients:** Blessed thistle contains various bioactive compounds, including sesquiterpene lactones (such as cnicin), flavonoids, tannins, and essential oils. These compounds are believed to contribute to the herb's medicinal properties, including its potential as a digestive tonic, appetite stimulant, and liver tonic.

**How to Prepare:** Blessed thistle is typically consumed as an herbal tea, tincture, or in supplement form (such as capsules or tablets). To make tea, dried blessed thistle leaves and flowers are steeped in hot water for several minutes before being strained and consumed.

**Dosage:** The appropriate dosage of blessed thistle can vary depending on factors such as age, health status, and the specific preparation being used. It's important to follow the recommended dosage on the product label or consult with a qualified herbalist or healthcare professional for personalized guidance.

**How to Use:** Blessed thistle tea, tincture, or supplements are typically taken orally. It's often used to support digestion, stimulate appetite, and promote liver health.

**Side Effects:** Blessed thistle is generally considered safe for most people when used in moderate amounts. However, some individuals may experience mild side effects such as gastrointestinal upset or allergic reactions. It may also interact with certain medications or have adverse effects in individuals with certain health conditions, such as hormone-sensitive conditions or bleeding disorders. Pregnant or breastfeeding individuals should consult with a healthcare professional before using blessed thistle supplements. It's important to use blessed thistle under the guidance of a healthcare professional and to discontinue use if any adverse effects occur.

**Cat's Claw:**

**Definition:** Cat's claw, scientifically known as Uncaria tomentosa, is a woody vine native to the Amazon rainforest and other parts of Central and South America. It has been used for centuries in traditional medicine by indigenous peoples for its potential health benefits.

**Ingredients:** Cat's claw contains various bioactive compounds, including alkaloids (such as oxindole alkaloids and quinovic acid glycosides), polyphenols, and other phytochemicals. These compounds are believed to contribute to the herb's medicinal properties, including its potential as an immune enhancer, anti-inflammatory, and antioxidant.

**How to Prepare:** Cat's claw is typically consumed as an herbal tea, tincture, or in supplement form (such as capsules or tablets). To make tea, dried cat's claw bark or leaves are steeped in hot water for several minutes before being strained and consumed.

**Dosage:** The appropriate dosage of cat's claw can vary depending on factors such as age, health status, and the specific preparation being used. It's important to follow the recommended dosage on the product label or consult with a qualified herbalist or healthcare professional for personalized guidance.

**How to Use:** Cat's claw tea, tincture, or supplements are typically taken orally. It's often used to support immune function, reduce inflammation, and promote overall well-being.

**Side Effects:** Cat's claw is generally considered safe for most people when used in moderate amounts. However, some individuals may experience mild side effects such as gastrointestinal upset or allergic reactions. It may also interact with certain medications or have adverse effects in individuals with certain health conditions, such as autoimmune diseases or bleeding disorders. Pregnant or breastfeeding individuals should consult with a healthcare professional before using cat's claw supplements. It's important to use cat's claw under the guidance of a healthcare professional and to discontinue use if any adverse effects occur.

**Chickweed:**

**Definition:** Chickweed, scientifically known as Stellaria media, is an annual herbaceous plant native to Europe but naturalized in many other parts of the world. It's often considered a common weed but has been used historically in traditional medicine for its potential health benefits.

**Ingredients:** Chickweed contains various bioactive compounds, including flavonoids, saponins, mucilage, and vitamins (such as vitamin C). These compounds are believed to contribute to the herb's medicinal properties, including its potential as a demulcent, anti-inflammatory, and mild diuretic.

**How to Prepare:** Chickweed is typically consumed as an herbal tea, infusion, or in fresh salads. To make tea, dried chickweed leaves and flowers are steeped in hot water for several minutes before being strained and consumed. It can also be used topically as a poultice or infused oil for skin conditions.

**Dosage:** The appropriate dosage of chickweed can vary depending on factors such as age, health status, and the specific preparation being used. It's important to follow the recommended dosage on the product label or consult with a qualified herbalist or healthcare professional for personalized guidance.

**How to Use:** Chickweed tea, infusion, or fresh leaves are typically taken orally. It's often used to soothe inflammation, support digestion, and promote overall well-being. Topically, chickweed can be applied to the skin to alleviate itching, irritation, or minor wounds.

**Side Effects:** Chickweed is generally considered safe for most people when consumed in moderate amounts. However, some individuals may experience allergic reactions or gastrointestinal upset. It may also interact with certain medications or have adverse effects in individuals with certain health conditions. Pregnant or breastfeeding individuals should consult with a healthcare professional before using chickweed supplements. It's important to use chickweed under the guidance of a healthcare professional and to discontinue use if any adverse effects occur.

**Cleavers:**

**Definition:** Cleavers, scientifically known as Galium aparine, is a herbaceous annual plant native to Europe, North America, Asia, and Australia. It has a long history of use in traditional medicine for its potential health benefits.

**Ingredients:** Cleavers contains various bioactive compounds, including iridoid glycosides, flavonoids, tannins, and mucilage. These compounds are believed to contribute to the herb's medicinal properties, including its potential as a diuretic, lymphatic tonic, and mild astringent.

**How to Prepare:** Cleavers is typically consumed as an herbal tea, infusion, or in fresh salads. To make tea, dried cleavers leaves and stems are steeped in hot water for several minutes before being strained and consumed. It can also be used topically as a poultice or infused oil for skin conditions.

**Dosage:** The appropriate dosage of cleavers can vary depending on factors such as age, health status, and the specific preparation being used. It's important to follow the recommended dosage on the product label or consult with a qualified herbalist or healthcare professional for personalized guidance.

**How to Use:** Cleavers tea, infusion, or fresh leaves are typically taken orally. It's often used to support lymphatic drainage, promote urinary tract health, and soothe inflammation. Topically, cleavers can be applied to the skin to alleviate itching, irritation, or minor wounds.

**Side Effects:** Cleavers is generally considered safe for most people when consumed in moderate amounts. However, some individuals may experience allergic reactions or gastrointestinal upset. It may also interact with certain medications or have adverse effects in individuals with certain health conditions. Pregnant or breastfeeding individuals should consult with a healthcare professional before using cleavers supplements. It's important to use cleavers under the guidance of a healthcare professional and to discontinue use if any adverse effects occur.

**Eucalyptus:**

**Definition:** Eucalyptus refers to a genus of flowering trees and shrubs, primarily native to Australia but also found in other parts of the world. Eucalyptus essential oil, extracted from the leaves of certain species, has a long history of use in traditional medicine for its potential health benefits.

**Ingredients:** Eucalyptus essential oil contains various bioactive compounds, including eucalyptol (cineole), terpenes, and flavonoids. These compounds are believed to contribute to the oil's medicinal properties, including its potential as an expectorant, decongestant, antiseptic, and anti-inflammatory.

**How to Prepare:** Eucalyptus essential oil can be used in aromatherapy, diffused in the air, or diluted and applied topically to the skin. It can also be added to steam inhalations or chest rubs to help relieve respiratory symptoms.

**Dosage:** The appropriate dosage of eucalyptus essential oil can vary depending on factors such as age, health status, and the specific application being used. It's important to follow the recommended dosage on the product label or consult with a qualified aromatherapist or healthcare professional for personalized guidance.

**How to Use:** Eucalyptus essential oil can be used aromatically, topically, or internally, depending on the intended application. It's often used to alleviate respiratory congestion, soothe sore muscles, promote relaxation, and support overall well-being.

**Side Effects:** Eucalyptus essential oil is generally considered safe for most people when used appropriately. However, it can be toxic if ingested in large amounts and should not be applied directly to the skin without proper dilution. Some individuals may experience allergic reactions or respiratory irritation when exposed to eucalyptus oil. It's important to use eucalyptus oil with caution, especially around children and pets. Pregnant or breastfeeding individuals should consult with a healthcare professional before using eucalyptus oil. If any adverse effects occur, discontinue use and seek medical attention.

**Feverfew:**

**Definition:** Feverfew, scientifically known as Tanacetum parthenium, is a perennial herb native to Europe but also found in other parts of the world. It has a long history of use in traditional medicine, particularly in European folk medicine, for its potential health benefits.

**Ingredients:** Feverfew contains various bioactive compounds, including sesquiterpene lactones (such as parthenolide), flavonoids, and volatile oils. These compounds are believed to contribute to the herb's medicinal properties, including its potential as an anti-inflammatory, analgesic, and migraine prophylactic.

**How to Prepare:** Feverfew is typically consumed as an herbal tea, tincture, or in supplement form (such as capsules or tablets). To make tea, dried feverfew leaves and flowers are steeped in hot water for several minutes before being strained and consumed.

**Dosage:** The appropriate dosage of feverfew can vary depending on factors such as age, health status, and the specific preparation being used. It's important to follow the recommended dosage on the product label or consult with a qualified herbalist or healthcare professional for personalized guidance.

**How to Use:** Feverfew tea, tincture, or supplements are typically taken orally. It's often used to alleviate headaches, including migraines, and to support overall well-being.

**Side Effects:** Feverfew is generally considered safe for most people when used in moderate amounts. However, some individuals may experience mild side effects such as gastrointestinal upset or allergic reactions. It may also interact with certain medications or have adverse effects in individuals with certain health conditions, such as bleeding disorders or pregnancy. It's important to use feverfew under the guidance of a healthcare professional and to discontinue use if any adverse effects occur.

**Ginseng:**

**Definition:** Ginseng refers to several species of perennial plants belonging to the Panax genus, including Panax ginseng (Asian ginseng) and Panax quinquefolius (American ginseng). Ginseng has been used for centuries in traditional medicine, particularly in East Asia, for its potential health benefits.

**Ingredients:** Ginseng root contains various bioactive compounds, including ginsenosides, polysaccharides, and peptides. These compounds are believed to contribute to the herb's medicinal properties, including its potential as an adaptogen, immune enhancer, and cognitive booster.

**How to Prepare:** Ginseng is typically consumed as a powdered root, herbal tea, tincture, or in supplement form (such as capsules or tablets). To make tea, dried ginseng root slices are simmered in water for several minutes before being strained and consumed.

**Dosage:** The appropriate dosage of ginseng can vary depending on factors such as age, health status, and the specific preparation being used. It's important to follow the recommended dosage on the product label or consult with a qualified herbalist or healthcare professional for personalized guidance.

**How to Use:** Ginseng powder, tea, tincture, or supplements are typically taken orally. It's often used to support energy levels, enhance cognitive function, and promote overall well-being.

**Side Effects:** Ginseng is generally considered safe for most people when used in moderate amounts. However, some individuals may experience mild side effects such as insomnia, gastrointestinal upset, or headaches. It may also interact with certain medications or have adverse effects in individuals with certain health conditions, such as high blood pressure or diabetes. Pregnant or breastfeeding individuals should consult with a healthcare professional before using ginseng supplements. It's important to use ginseng under the guidance of a healthcare professional and to discontinue use if any adverse effects occur.

**Goldenseal:**

**Definition:** Goldenseal, scientifically known as Hydrastis canadensis, is a perennial herb native to North America. It has a long history of use in traditional Native American medicine and later in folk medicine for its potential health benefits.

**Ingredients:** Goldenseal root contains various bioactive compounds, including alkaloids (such as berberine and hydrastine), flavonoids, and volatile oils. These compounds are believed to contribute to the herb's medicinal properties, including its potential as an antimicrobial, anti-inflammatory, and immune enhancer.

**How to Prepare:** Goldenseal is typically consumed as an herbal tea, tincture, or in supplement form (such as capsules or tablets). To make tea, dried goldenseal root or leaves are steeped in hot water for several minutes before being strained and consumed.

**Dosage:** The appropriate dosage of goldenseal can vary depending on factors such as age, health status, and the specific preparation being used. It's important to follow the recommended dosage on the product label or consult with a qualified herbalist or healthcare professional for personalized guidance.

**How to Use:** Goldenseal tea, tincture, or supplements are typically taken orally. It's often used to support immune function, promote digestive health, and soothe inflammation.

**Side Effects:** Goldenseal is generally considered safe for most people when used in moderate amounts. However, some individuals may experience mild side effects such as gastrointestinal upset or allergic reactions. It may also interact with certain medications or have adverse effects in individuals with certain health conditions, such as high blood pressure or pregnancy. It's important to use goldenseal under the guidance of a healthcare professional and to discontinue use if any adverse effects occur.

**Hops:**

**Definition:** Hops, scientifically known as Humulus lupulus, is a perennial climbing vine native to Europe, Asia, and North America. It is primarily known for its use in brewing beer but has also been used historically in traditional medicine for its potential health benefits.

**Ingredients:** Hops flowers contain various bioactive compounds, including bitter acids (such as humulone and lupulone), essential oils, flavonoids, and polyphenols. These compounds are believed to contribute to the herb's medicinal properties, including its potential as a sedative, relaxant, and digestive aid.

**How to Prepare:** Hops is typically consumed as an herbal tea, tincture, or in supplement form (such as capsules or tablets). To make tea, dried hops flowers are steeped in hot water for several minutes before being strained and consumed.

**Dosage:** The appropriate dosage of hops can vary depending on factors such as age, health status, and the specific preparation being used. It's important to follow the recommended dosage on the product label or consult with a qualified herbalist or healthcare professional for personalized guidance.

**How to Use:** Hops tea, tincture, or supplements are typically taken orally. It's often used to promote relaxation, relieve anxiety, and support sleep.

**Side Effects:** Hops is generally considered safe for most people when used in moderate amounts. However, some individuals may experience mild side effects such as drowsiness, gastrointestinal upset, or allergic reactions. It may also interact with certain medications or have adverse effects in individuals with certain health conditions, such as depression or hormone-sensitive conditions. It's important to use hops under the guidance of a healthcare professional and to discontinue use if any adverse effects occur.

**Bio Ferro Tonic:**

**Definition:** Bio Ferro Tonic is a dietary supplement primarily composed of herbs and minerals. It's often marketed as a natural way to support overall health, particularly by promoting blood health and circulation.

**Ingredients:** Typical ingredients in Bio Ferro Tonic may include a blend of herbs such as burdock root, yellow dock root, sarsaparilla root, and cascara sagrada bark, along with minerals like iron and potassium phosphate.

**How to Prepare:** Bio Ferro Tonic usually comes in liquid form and is typically taken orally. It's important to follow the instructions on the product label for dosage and administration.

**Dosage:** The dosage can vary depending on the specific product and individual needs. It's crucial to consult with a healthcare professional or follow the recommended dosage on the product label to avoid potential side effects.

**How to Use:** Bio Ferro Tonic is often taken by adding the recommended dosage to water or juice and consuming it orally. It's important to shake the bottle well before use and store it according to the manufacturer's instructions.

**Side Effects:** While Bio Ferro Tonic is generally considered safe when used as directed, some individuals may experience side effects such as digestive discomfort, allergic reactions, or interactions with medications. It's essential to consult with a healthcare provider before starting any new supplement regimen, especially if you have underlying health conditions or are taking medications.

**Bladderwrack:**

**Definition:** Bladderwrack is a type of seaweed or marine algae commonly used in traditional medicine and as a dietary supplement. It's known for its potential health benefits, particularly related to thyroid health and weight management.

**Ingredients:** Bladderwrack contains various nutrients, including iodine, vitamins, minerals, and antioxidants. The primary active components are iodine and fucoidan, a type of carbohydrate found in brown seaweeds.

**How to Prepare:** Bladderwrack supplements are available in various forms, including capsules, powders, and liquid extracts. They can be taken orally with water or added to smoothies and other beverages.

**Dosage:** The appropriate dosage of bladderwrack can vary based on factors such as age, health status, and the specific product being used. It's essential to follow the recommended dosage on the product label or consult with a healthcare professional for personalized guidance.

**How to Use:** Bladderwrack supplements are typically taken orally, either with water or mixed into food or beverages. It's important to follow the instructions on the product label and avoid exceeding the recommended dosage.

**Side Effects:** While bladderwrack is generally considered safe for most people when used in moderation, excessive intake of iodine from bladderwrack supplements can cause thyroid dysfunction and other adverse effects. Individuals with thyroid disorders, iodine sensitivity, or certain medical conditions should exercise caution and consult with a healthcare provider before using bladderwrack supplements. Common side effects may include digestive upset, allergic reactions, or interactions with medications.

**Blood Purifier:**

**Definition:** Blood purifiers are herbal remedies or dietary supplements believed to cleanse or detoxify the blood, often promoting overall health and well-being. They are thought to support the body's natural detoxification processes and improve blood circulation.

**Ingredients:** Blood purifiers may contain a variety of herbs and botanical extracts known for their purported cleansing and detoxifying properties. Common ingredients include burdock root, red clover, dandelion root, and yellow dock root, among others.

**How to Prepare:** Blood purifiers are typically available in various forms, including capsules, tablets, powders, and liquid extracts. They are usually taken orally with water or juice, following the recommended dosage on the product label.

**Dosage:** The dosage of blood purifiers can vary depending on the specific product and individual needs. It's important to adhere to the recommended dosage on the product label or consult with a healthcare professional for personalized guidance.

**How to Use:** Blood purifiers are typically taken orally, either with water or mixed into beverages. They are often used as part of a detoxification regimen or to support overall health and vitality.

**Side Effects:** While blood purifiers are generally considered safe for most people when used as directed, some individuals may experience side effects such as digestive discomfort, allergic reactions, or interactions with medications. It's important to consult with a healthcare provider before starting any new supplement regimen, especially if you have underlying health conditions or are taking medications.

**Blue Vervain:**

**Definition:** Blue vervain, also known as Verbena hastata, is a perennial herb native to North America. It has been used in traditional medicine for centuries to treat various ailments, including anxiety, insomnia, and digestive issues.

**Ingredients:** Blue vervain contains several active compounds, including aucubin, verbenalin, and volatile oils. These compounds are believed to contribute to the herb's medicinal properties.

**How to Prepare:** Blue vervain is typically consumed as a tea or tincture. To make tea, dried blue vervain leaves and flowers are steeped in hot water for several minutes before being strained and consumed. Tinctures are prepared by steeping the herb in alcohol or vinegar to extract its active compounds.

**Dosage:** The appropriate dosage of blue vervain can vary depending on factors such as age, health status, and the specific preparation being used. It's important to follow the recommended dosage on the product label or consult with a qualified herbalist or healthcare professional for personalized guidance.

**How to Use:** Blue vervain tea or tincture is typically taken orally. It can be consumed on its own or mixed with honey or other herbal teas for added flavor.

**Side Effects:** While blue vervain is generally considered safe for most people when used in moderation, excessive intake may cause digestive upset or allergic reactions in some individuals. Pregnant or breastfeeding women should avoid blue vervain due to its potential to stimulate uterine contractions. As with any herbal remedy, it's important to consult with a healthcare provider before using blue vervain, especially if you have underlying health conditions or are taking medications.

**Bromide Plus Powder:**

**Definition:** Bromide Plus Powder is a dietary supplement formulated to support thyroid health and promote overall well-being. It typically contains a blend of herbs and minerals that are believed to have beneficial effects on thyroid function.

**Ingredients:** Bromide Plus Powder often contains a combination of herbs such as bladderwrack, sea moss, and burdock root, along with minerals like iodine and potassium phosphate. These ingredients are thought to support thyroid function and maintain optimal iodine levels in the body.

**How to Prepare:** Bromide Plus Powder is usually mixed with water or juice to create a drinkable solution. It's important to follow the instructions on the product label for dosage and preparation.

**Dosage:** The dosage of Bromide Plus Powder can vary depending on the specific product and individual needs. It's crucial to consult with a healthcare professional or follow the recommended dosage on the product label to avoid potential side effects.

**How to Use:** Bromide Plus Powder is typically taken orally by mixing the recommended dosage with water or juice. It's important to shake or stir the mixture well before consuming it to ensure even distribution of the ingredients.

**Side Effects:** While Bromide Plus Powder is generally considered safe when used as directed, some individuals may experience side effects such as digestive discomfort or allergic reactions to certain ingredients. It's essential to consult with a healthcare provider before starting any new supplement regimen, especially if you have underlying health conditions or are taking medications.

**Bugleweed:**

**Definition:** Bugleweed, also known as Lycopusvirginicus, is a perennial herb native to North America and Europe. It has been used in traditional medicine to treat various conditions, including hyperthyroidism, anxiety, and insomnia.

**Ingredients:** Bugleweed contains several active compounds, including lithospermic acid, phenolic acids, and flavonoids. These compounds are believed to contribute to the herb's medicinal properties, particularly its ability to regulate thyroid function.

**How to Prepare:** Bugleweed is commonly consumed as a tea or tincture. To make tea, dried bugleweed leaves and flowers are steeped in hot water for several minutes before being strained and consumed. Tinctures are prepared by steeping the herb in alcohol or vinegar to extract its active compounds.

**Dosage:** The appropriate dosage of bugleweed can vary depending on factors such as age, health status, and the specific preparation being used. It's important to follow the recommended dosage on the product label or consult with a qualified herbalist or healthcare professional for personalized guidance.

**How to Use:** Bugleweed tea or tincture is typically taken orally. It can be consumed on its own or mixed with honey or other herbal teas for added flavor.

**Side Effects:** While bugleweed is generally considered safe for most people when used in moderation, excessive intake may cause digestive upset or allergic reactions in some individuals. Pregnant or breastfeeding women should avoid bugleweed due to its potential to stimulate uterine contractions. As with any herbal remedy, it's important to consult with a healthcare provider before using bugleweed, especially if you have underlying health conditions or are taking medications.

**Burdock:**

**Definition:** Burdock, scientifically known as Arctium lappa, is a biennial plant native to Europe and Asia but now found worldwide. It's part of the Asteraceae family and has been used for centuries in traditional medicine and culinary practices.

**Ingredients:** Burdock contains various nutrients, including carbohydrates, fiber, vitamins (such as vitamin B6, folate, and vitamin C), and minerals (including potassium, magnesium, and manganese). It also contains active compounds such as polyphenols and volatile oils.

**How to Prepare:** Burdock can be prepared and consumed in various ways. The roots, leaves, and seeds are all utilized for different purposes. The root is commonly used in cooking, herbal teas, tinctures, and supplements, while the leaves and seeds are sometimes used in herbal preparations.

**Dosage:** The appropriate dosage of burdock root can vary depending on the specific form and intended use. For culinary purposes, there are no strict dosage guidelines, but for supplements or herbal remedies, it's essential to follow the recommended dosage on the product label or consult with a healthcare professional.

**How to Use:** Burdock root can be used in cooking by peeling, slicing, and adding it to soups, stews, stir-fries, or salads. It can also be brewed into a tea or used to make tinctures or extracts for medicinal purposes. Some people may also take burdock root supplements in capsule or powder form.

**Side Effects:** While burdock is generally considered safe for most people when consumed in moderate amounts, some individuals may experience allergic reactions or digestive upset. Additionally, burdock may interact with certain medications or have adverse effects in individuals with certain health conditions, such as diabetes or allergies to plants in the Asteraceae family. It's important to consult with a healthcare provider before using burdock, especially if you have underlying health conditions or are taking medications.

**Cascara Sagrada:**

**Definition:** Cascara Sagrada, scientifically known as Rhamnus purshiana, is a species of buckthorn native to western North America. It has been used traditionally as a laxative and to promote bowel regularity.

**Ingredients:** The primary active ingredients in cascara sagrada are anthraquinone glycosides, particularly cascarosides A and B. These compounds stimulate peristalsis in the colon, leading to increased bowel movements.

**How to Prepare:** Cascara sagrada is typically prepared as an herbal tea, tincture, or capsule. To make tea, dried cascara sagrada bark is steeped in hot water for several minutes before being strained and consumed. Tinctures are prepared by steeping the bark in alcohol to extract its active compounds.

**Dosage:** The appropriate dosage of cascara sagrada can vary depending on the specific preparation and intended use. It's important to follow the recommended dosage on the product label or consult with a healthcare professional for personalized guidance.

**How to Use:** Cascara sagrada tea or tincture is typically taken orally. It's important to start with a low dose and gradually increase if needed to avoid potential side effects such as cramping or diarrhea.

**Side Effects:** Cascara sagrada is considered safe for short-term use when used as directed. However, long-term or excessive use may lead to dependence, electrolyte imbalance, or dehydration. It may also interact with certain medications or have adverse effects in individuals with certain health conditions. It's important to use cascara sagrada under the guidance of a healthcare professional and to discontinue use if any adverse effects occur.

**Cell Food:**

**Definition:** Cell Food is a dietary supplement marketed as a highly oxygenating and alkalizing formula. It's claimed to support overall health and vitality by providing essential nutrients and oxygen to the cells.

**Ingredients:** The exact ingredients of Cell Food can vary depending on the brand, but it typically contains a proprietary blend of minerals, enzymes, electrolytes, and trace elements. Some common ingredients may include purified water, dissolved oxygen, seawater extract, and plant-based enzymes.

**How to Prepare:** Cell Food is usually available in liquid form and is typically taken orally. It can be consumed directly or diluted in water or juice before consumption.

**Dosage:** The dosage of Cell Food can vary depending on the specific product and individual needs. It's important to follow the recommended dosage on the product label or consult with a healthcare professional for personalized guidance.

**How to Use:** Cell Food is typically taken orally, either directly or mixed into water or juice. It's important to shake the bottle well before use and to store it according to the manufacturer's instructions.

**Side Effects:** Cell Food is generally considered safe for most people when used as directed. However, some individuals may experience mild digestive upset or allergic reactions to certain ingredients. It's essential to consult with a healthcare provider before starting any new supplement regimen, especially if you have underlying health conditions or are taking medications.

**Chaparral:**

**Definition:** Chaparral, scientifically known as Larrea tridentata, is a shrub native to the southwestern United States and northern

Mexico. It has been used for centuries by Native American tribes for its medicinal properties and is commonly used in herbal medicine today.

**Ingredients:** Chaparral contains several bioactive compounds, including nordihydroguaiaretic acid (NDGA), flavonoids, lignans, and volatile oils. NDGA is believed to be the primary active compound responsible for many of chaparral's therapeutic effects.

**How to Prepare:** Chaparral can be prepared and consumed in various forms, including teas, tinctures, capsules, and topical preparations. To make tea, dried chaparral leaves are steeped in hot water for several minutes before being strained and consumed. Tinctures are prepared by steeping the herb in alcohol or vinegar to extract its active compounds.

**Dosage:** The appropriate dosage of chaparral can vary depending on the specific form and intended use. It's important to follow the recommended dosage on the product label or consult with a healthcare professional for personalized guidance.

**How to Use:** Chaparral tea or tincture is typically taken orally. It can also be applied topically to the skin for certain conditions. It's important to use chaparral products as directed and to discontinue use if any adverse effects occur.

**Side Effects:** Chaparral is generally considered safe for most people when used in moderate amounts. However, excessive intake or prolonged use may lead to liver toxicity or other adverse effects. It may also interact with certain medications or have adverse effects in individuals with certain health conditions. It's important to use chaparral under the guidance of a healthcare professional and to discontinue use if any adverse effects occur.

**Kelp:**

**Definition:** Kelp refers to several species of large brown algae belonging to the Laminariales order. It is commonly found in underwater forests along rocky coastlines around the world. Kelp has been used for centuries in various cultures, particularly in East Asia, for its nutritional and medicinal properties.

**Ingredients:** Kelp is rich in various nutrients, including iodine, vitamins (such as vitamin K, vitamin C, and B vitamins), minerals (including calcium, magnesium, and potassium), antioxidants, and fiber. These nutrients are believed to contribute to the seaweed's potential health benefits, including its role in thyroid function, bone health, and immune support.

**How to Prepare:** Kelp is typically consumed dried, powdered, or in supplement form (such as capsules or tablets). It can also be used in cooking, particularly in soups, salads, and stir-fries. Kelp supplements are available in various forms, including powdered extracts, tablets, and liquid extracts.

**Dosage:** The appropriate dosage of kelp can vary depending on factors such as age, health status, and the specific preparation being used. It's important to follow the recommended dosage on the product label or consult with a qualified healthcare professional for personalized guidance.

**How to Use:** Kelp supplements are typically taken orally with water. They can be consumed as part of a daily nutritional regimen to support overall health and well-being. Kelp can also be incorporated into recipes as a flavorful and nutritious ingredient.

**Side Effects:** While kelp is generally considered safe for most people when consumed in moderate amounts, excessive intake of iodine-rich foods or supplements, including kelp, can lead to thyroid dysfunction or iodine toxicity. Some individuals may also be allergic to seaweed and experience allergic reactions. Pregnant or breastfeeding individuals should consult with a healthcare professional before using kelp supplements. It's important to use kelp under the guidance of a healthcare professional and to discontinue use if any adverse effects occur.

**Agrimony:**

**Definition:** Agrimony, scientifically known as Agrimonia eupatoria, is a perennial herbaceous plant native to Europe, Asia, and North America. It has a long history of use in traditional medicine, particularly in European folk medicine, for its potential health benefits.

**Ingredients:** Agrimony contains various bioactive compounds, including tannins, flavonoids, phenolic acids, and volatile oils. These compounds are believed to contribute to the herb's medicinal properties, including its potential as an astringent, anti-inflammatory, and digestive aid.

**How to Prepare:** Agrimony is typically prepared and consumed as an herbal tea, tincture, or poultice. To make tea, dried agrimony leaves and flowers are steeped in hot water for several minutes before being strained and consumed. Tinctures are prepared by steeping the herb in alcohol or vinegar to extract its active compounds.

**Dosage:** The appropriate dosage of agrimony can vary depending on factors such as age, health status, and the specific preparation being used. It's important to follow the recommended dosage on the product label or consult with a qualified herbalist or healthcare professional for personalized guidance.

**How to Use:** Agrimony tea, tincture, or poultice is typically taken orally or applied topically. It's often consumed to soothe gastrointestinal issues, such as indigestion and diarrhea, or used externally to treat skin conditions.

**Side Effects:** Agrimony is generally considered safe for most people when used in moderate amounts. However, some individuals may experience allergic reactions or gastrointestinal upset. It may also interact with certain medications or have adverse effects in individuals with certain health conditions. It's important to use agrimony under the guidance of a healthcare professional and to discontinue use if any adverse effects occur.

## Alfalfa:

**Definition:** Alfalfa, scientifically known as Medicago sativa, is a flowering plant in the pea family native to Asia but cultivated worldwide. It's primarily grown as fodder for livestock, but it has also been used in traditional medicine for its potential health benefits.

**Ingredients:** Alfalfa contains various bioactive compounds, including vitamins (such as vitamin A, vitamin C, and vitamin K), minerals (including calcium, magnesium, and potassium), amino acids, and phytoestrogens. These compounds are believed to contribute to the herb's medicinal properties, including its potential as a nutritive tonic, diuretic, and hormone balancer.

**How to Prepare:** Alfalfa is typically consumed as sprouts, herbal tea, or in supplement form (such as capsules or tablets). To make tea, dried alfalfa leaves are steeped in hot water for several minutes before being strained and consumed.

**Dosage:** The appropriate dosage of alfalfa can vary depending on factors such as age, health status, and the specific preparation being used. It's important to follow the recommended dosage on the product label or consult with a qualified herbalist or healthcare professional for personalized guidance.

**How to Use:** Alfalfa sprouts, tea, or supplements are typically taken orally. It's often consumed as a dietary supplement to support overall health and well-being, as well as to promote kidney health and hormone balance.

**Side Effects:** Alfalfa is generally considered safe for most people when consumed in moderate amounts. However, some individuals may experience allergic reactions or digestive upset. It may also interact with certain medications or have adverse effects in individuals with certain health conditions, such as autoimmune diseases or hormone-sensitive conditions. Pregnant or breastfeeding individuals should consult with a healthcare professional before using alfalfa supplements. It's important to use alfalfa under the guidance of a healthcare professional and to discontinue use if any adverse effects occur.

# THE END

www.ingramcontent.com/pod-product-compliance
Lightning Source LLC
Chambersburg PA
CBHW081558250726
48653CB00009B/3495